C000219679

# CONGRATULATIONS YOU'RE A MUM

*Kate Freeman*

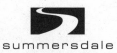

summersdale

CONGRATULATIONS YOU'RE A MUM

Summersdale Publishers Ltd
46 West Street
Chichester
West Sussex
PO19 1RP
UK

www.summersdale.com

Printed and bound in China

ISBN: 978-1-84953-746-9

Substantial discounts on bulk quantities of Summersdale books are available to corporations, professional associations and other organisations. For details contact Nicky Douglas by telephone: +44 (0) 1243 756902, fax: +44 (0) 1243 786300 or email: nicky@summersdale.com.

To........Jena........

Love
From.....All at N° 45....

x

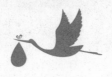

# Life began with waking up and loving my mother's face.

*George Eliot*

# Think of stretch marks as pregnancy service stripes.

*Joyce Armor*

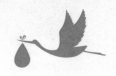

When my baby was born... I suddenly was so full of love that it was a little bit as if I was drugged.

*Anne-Marie Duff*

**A baby is born
with a need to be
loved – and never
outgrows it.**

*Frank A. Clark*

# IT'S 3 A.M. AGAIN!

**Babies are always more trouble than you thought – and more wonderful.**

*Charles Osgood*

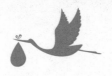

If the choice is
between sleeping
and the housework,
sleep.

*Anonymous*

**A mother always has to think twice, once for herself and once for her child.**

*Sophia Loren*

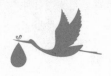

**There never was a child so lovely, but his mother was glad to get him asleep.**

*Ralph Waldo Emerson*

# A man's work is from sun to sun, but a mother's work is never done.

*Anonymous*

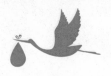

There is no way to
be a perfect mother,
and a million ways
to be a good one.

*Jill Churchill*

# SMALL IS BEAUTIFUL.

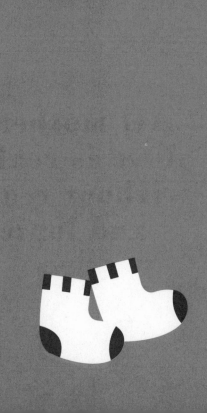

# All motherly love is really without reason and logic.

Joan Chen

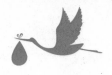

# When they placed you in my arms, you slipped into my heart.

*Anonymous*

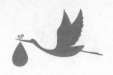

**Aside from new babies, new mothers must be the most beautiful creatures on earth.**

*Terri Guillemets*

Having a baby is like falling in love again, both with your husband and your child.

*Tina Brown*

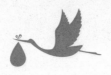

# For when a child is born the mother also is born again.

Gilbert Parker

**Think of your
mother and smile
for all of the good
precious moments.**

*Ana Monnar*

# TIME FOR ENDLESS CUDDLES AND KISSES.

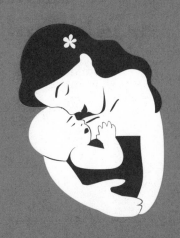

# We made a
# wish and you
# came true.

*Anonymous*

**Birth is an experience that demonstrates that life is not merely function and utility, but form and beauty.**

*Christopher Largen*

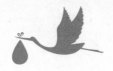

# There is a power that comes to women when they give birth.

*Sheryl Feldman*

# A grand adventure is about to begin.

*A. A. Milne*

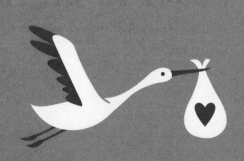

# LOOK WHAT THE STORK BROUGHT!

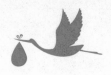

# Babies are such a nice way to start people.

*Don Herold*

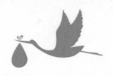

**Childbirth classes neglect to teach one critical skill: how to breathe, count and swear all at the same time.**

Linda Fiterman

**Making the decision
to have a child is
momentous. It is
to decide forever
to have your heart
go walking around
outside your body.**

*Elizabeth Stone*

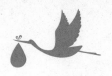

A new baby is like
the beginning of all
things – wonder,
hope, a dream of
possibilities.

*Eda LeShan*

It seems to
me my mother
was the most
splendid woman
I ever knew.

*Charlie Chaplin*

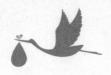

# A mother's arms are made of tenderness and children sleep soundly in them.

*Victor Hugo*

**Loving a baby is a circular business... the more you give the more you get.**

*Penelope Leach*

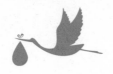

There is no
velvet so soft as
a mother's lap, no
rose as lovely as
her smile, no path
so flowery as that
imprinted with
her footsteps.

*Edward Thomson*

**Motherhood is at its best when the tender chords of sympathy have been touched.**

*Paul Harris*

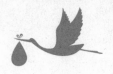

# There's nothing like a mama-hug.

*Adabella Radici*

# WHO'S GOT A BEAUTIFUL SMILE?

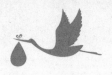

# There is only one pretty child in the world, and every mother has it.

*Chinese proverb*

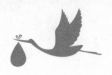

# The only love that I really believe in is a mother's love for her children.

*Karl Lagerfeld*

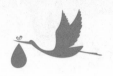

The heart of a
mother is a deep
abyss at the bottom
of which you
will always find
forgiveness.

*Honoré de Balzac*

If evolution
really works, how
come mothers only
have two hands?

*Milton Berle*

# A mother's love for her child is like nothing else in the world.

*Agatha Christie*

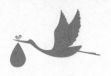

**Behind all your
stories is always
your mother's story,
because hers is
where yours begins.**

*Mitch Albom*

# I THINK IT'S NAP TIME.

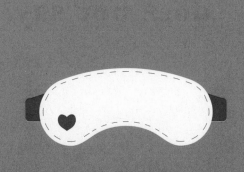

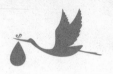

# A mother understands what a child does not say.

*Jewish proverb*

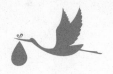

Our mothers
always remain the
strangest, craziest
people we've
ever met.

*Marguerite Duras*

Womanliness means only motherhood; all love begins and ends there.

*Robert Browning*

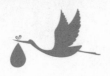

# Mother is the one we count on for the things that matter most of all.

*Katharine Butler Hathaway*

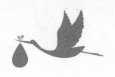

**Motherhood in
all its guises and
permutations is
more art than
science.**

Melinda M. Marshall

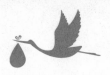

For the hand that
rocks the cradle is
the hand that rules
the world.

*William Ross Wallace*

# SHAKE, RATTLE AND ROLL!

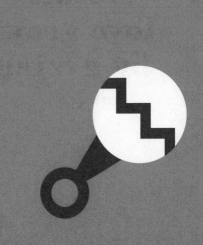

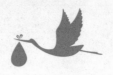

# Mother's love grows by giving.

Charles Lamb

My mother
made a brilliant
impression upon my
childhood life. She
shone for me like
the evening star.

*Winston Churchill*

# Most mothers are instinctive philosophers.

*Harriet Beecher Stowe*

**Mother's love is peace. It need not be acquired, it need not be deserved.**

Erich Fromm

My mother's great...
She could stop
you from doing
anything, through
a closed door even,
with a single look.

*Whoopi Goldberg*

**Mother is the heartbeat in the home; and without her, there seems to be no heart throb.**

*Leroy Brownlow*

# TIME
## FOR YOUR
## CLOSE-UP.

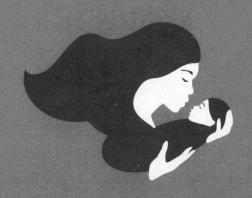

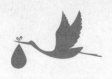

**No language can express the power and beauty and heroism of a mother's love.**

*Edwin H. Chapin*

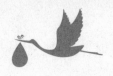

**Mother is the name for God in the lips and hearts of little children.**

*William Makepeace Thackeray*

If love is
sweet as a flower,
then my mother is
that sweet flower
of love.

Stevie Wonder

When you look at
your mother, you
are looking at the
purest love you
will ever know.

*Mitch Albom*

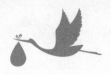

**All mothers are
rich when they love
their children...
there are no poor
mothers, no ugly
ones, no old ones.**

*Maurice Maeterlinck*

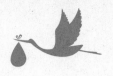

# Children are the anchors that hold a mother to life.

*Sophocles*

# SLEEP?
## WHAT'S THAT?

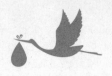

# Children are not a distraction from more important work. They are the most important work.

*C. S. Lewis*

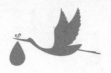

**Any mother could perform the jobs of several air traffic controllers with ease.**

*Lisa Alther*

**Motherhood has a very humanising effect. Everything gets reduced to essentials.**

*Meryl Streep*

**God could not be everywhere, so he created mothers.**

Jewish proverb

# What is a home without children? Quiet.

*Henny Youngman*

Mother love is the
fuel that enables
a normal human
being to do the
impossible.

*Marion C. Garretty*

# LET'S PLAY!

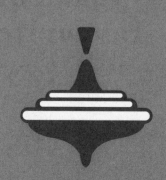

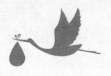

# You will always be your child's favourite toy.

*Vicki Lansky*

# No animal is so inexhaustible as an excited infant.

Amy Leslie

**A mother's arms are more comforting than anyone else's.**

*Diana, Princess of Wales*

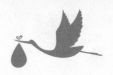

**Children keep us
in check. Their
laughter prevents
our hearts from
hardening.**

Queen Rania of Jordan

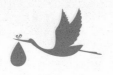

# While we try to teach our children all about life, our children teach us what life is all about.

*Angela Schwindt*

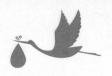

**A mother is not
a person to lean
on but a person
to make leaning
unnecessary.**

*Dorothy Canfield Fisher*

# FUN
# PLUS
# ONE.

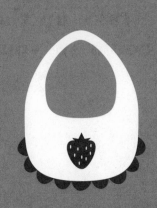

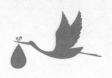

**Sometimes... the
smallest things
take up the most
room in your heart.**

*A. A. Milne*

# My mother
# is a walking
# miracle.

Leonardo DiCaprio

**All mothers are
quintessential: in
pain and joy they
are always with
us, encouraging,
instructing, loving.**

*Peter Megargee Brown*

The most
beautiful word
on the lips of
mankind is the
word 'Mother'.

Kahlil Gibran

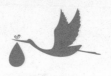

I shall never
forget my mother,
for it was she
who planted and
nurtured the first
seeds of good
within me.

*Immanuel Kant*

# When you are a mother, you are never really alone in your thoughts.

Sophia Loren

# ONE FOR
## THE FAMILY
# ALBUM.

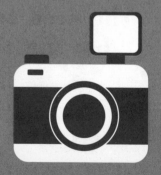

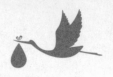

**I understood
once I held a baby
in my arms, why
some people have
the need to keep
having them.**

Spalding Gray

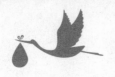

# Of all the rights of women, the greatest is to be a mother.

*Lin Yutang*

The most
consistent gift
and burden of
motherhood
is advice.

Susan Chira

**A mother is she
who can take the
place of all others
but whose place no
one else can take.**

*Gaspard Mermillod*

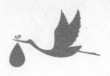

**Children and mothers never truly part – bound in the beating of each other's heart.**

*Charlotte Gray*

There is no
reciprocity. Men love
women, women love
children. Children
love hamsters.

*Alice Thomas Ellis*

# HERE COMES THE AEROPLANE!

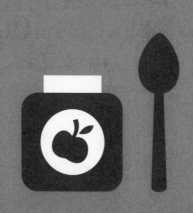

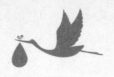

**Don't ever tell
the mother of a
newborn that her
baby's smile is
just gas.**

*Jill Woodhull*

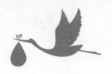

# Mothers are the heart of any household.

*Helena Bonham Carter*

# A mother...
seeing there are
only four pieces of
pie for five people,
promptly announces
she never did
care for pie.

*Tenneva Jordan*

**Sometimes the strength of motherhood is greater than natural laws.**

Barbara Kingsolver

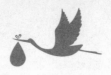

**A little girl, asked where her home was, replied, 'Where Mother is.'**

*Keith L. Brooks*

# Men are what their mothers made them.

Ralph Waldo Emerson

# GOODBYE
# LIE-INS.

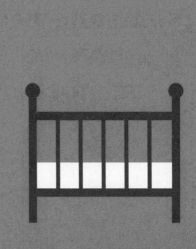

# It takes someone really brave to be a mother.

*Anonymous*

**There's no road map on how to raise a family: it's always an enormous negotiation.**

*Meryl Streep*

# Mother is a verb,
# not a noun.

*Proverb*

# Where there is a mother in the home, matters go well.

*Amos Bronson Alcott*

# The natural state of motherhood is unselfishness.

Jessica Lange

The patience of a
mother might be
likened to a tube
of toothpaste – it's
never quite all gone.

*Anonymous*

# SAY HELLO TO YOUR NEW LIFE AS 'MUM!'

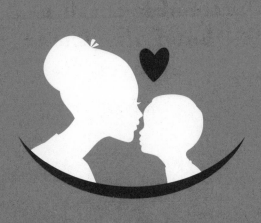

# My mother had a great deal of trouble with me, but I think she enjoyed it.

*Mark Twain*

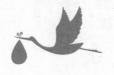

# In a child's eyes, a mother is a goddess.

*N. K. Jemisin*

There are
only two lasting
bequests we can
hope to give our
children. One of
these is roots. The
other, wings.

*Hodding Carter*

**No influence is
so powerful as that
of the mother.**

Sarah Josepha Hale

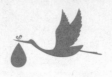

The best way to
keep children at
home is to make the
home atmosphere
pleasant, and let the
air out of the tyres.

*Dorothy Parker*

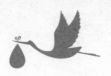

Stories first heard
at a mother's knee
are never wholly
forgotten.

Giovanni Ruffini

# YOU ARE
# THE NEW
# ENCYCLOPEDIA.

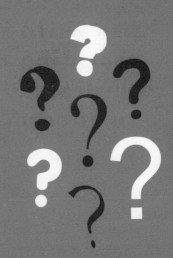

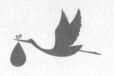

# The raising of a child is the building of a cathedral. You can't cut corners.

*Dave Eggers*

# A smart mother makes often a better diagnosis than a poor doctor.

*August Bier*

# A mother's heart is the child's classroom.

*Henry Ward Beecher*

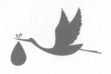

If you can
give your son or
daughter only
one gift, let it be
enthusiasm.

*Bruce Barton*

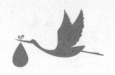

**Mother – that was
the bank where we
deposited all our
hurts and worries.**

*Thomas De Witt Talmage*

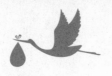

# All that I am
# my mother
# made me.

*John Quincy Adams*

# LIFE'S A WALK IN THE PARK.

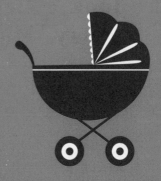

# Nothing beats having this beautiful child look at me and say, 'Mum'.

*Nicole Appleton*

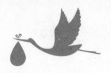

She never quite
leaves her children
at home, even when
she doesn't take
them along.

*Margaret Culkin Banning*

# Mothers always know.

*Oprah Winfrey*

To a child's ear,
'mother' is magic
in any language.

*Arlene Benedict*

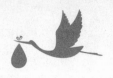

# The art of mothering is to teach the art of living to children.

Elaine Heffner

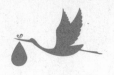

**Mum always says
the right thing.
She always makes
everything better.**

*Sophie Kinsella*

# YOU'RE THE BEST MUM IN THE WORLD!

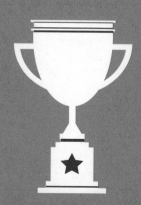

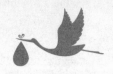

# There was never a great man who had not a great mother.

Olive Schreiner

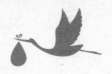

# A father's goodness is higher than the mountain, a mother's deeper than the sea.

*Japanese proverb*

**An ounce of
mother is worth
a ton of priest.**

*Spanish proverb*

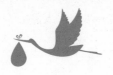

**All that I am
or ever hope to
be, I owe to my
angel mother.**

*Abraham Lincoln*

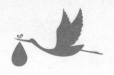

When a child needs
a mother to talk to,
nobody else but a
mother will do.

*Erica Jong*

Mothers... speak
the same tongue.
A mother in
Manchuria could
converse with a
mother in Nebraska
and never miss
a word.

*Will Rogers*

# HERE'S TO YOUR NEW ADVENTURE!

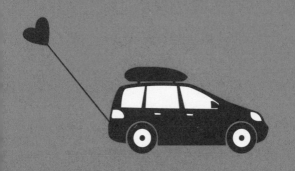

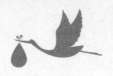

**A suburban
mother's role is
to deliver children
obstetrically
once, and by car
forever after.**

*Peter De Vries*

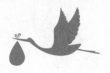

I know enough to know that when you're in a pickle... call Mom.

Jennifer Garner

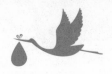

# A mother holds her children's hands for a short while, but their hearts for ever.

*Anonymous*

# A mother is the truest friend we have.

*Washington Irving*

If you're interested in
finding out more about our
books, find us on Facebook at
Summersdale Publishers and
follow us on Twitter at
@Summersdale.

www.summersdale.com